Klaus Kaufmann, DSc and Anne

Making
Sauerkraut
and pickled vegetables at home

Creative recipes for
lactic-fermented food
to improve your health

books
Alive

Summertown
Tennessee

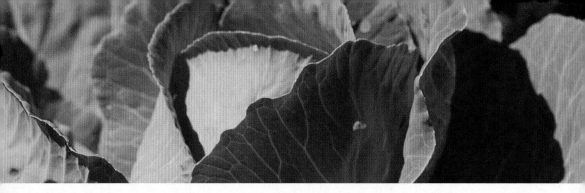

Contents

All About Sauerkraut

Note: Conversions in this book (from imperial to metric) are not exact. They have been rounded to the nearest measurement for convenience. Exact measurements are given in imperial. The recipes in this book are by no means to be taken as therapeutic. They simply promote the philosophy of both the author and alive Books in relation to whole foods, health and nutrition, while incorporating the practical advice given by the author in the first section of the book.

Sauerkraut Recipes

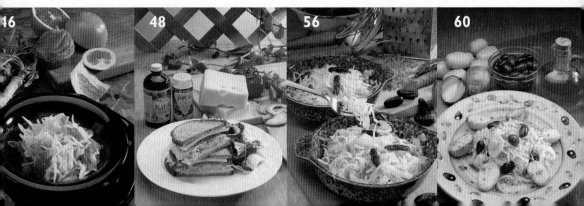

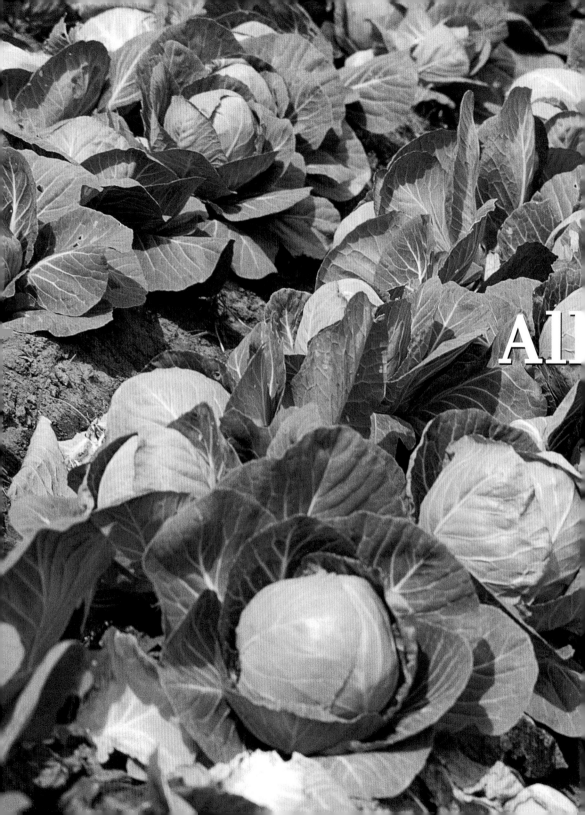

All

About Sauerkraut

Lactic-acid fermentation
–The ancient and proven
preservation method–
rediscovered!

Introduction ·

The growing health and natural lifestyle movement is beginning to rediscover the simple remedies and healing agents found in fresh, raw fruits and vegetables. Yet, at the same time, an opposing and seemingly greater force is pushing more and more consumers in the direction of frozen and processed foods, which have more than tripled their sales in Canada and the United States over the past decade. The public, in its continuous search for convenience meals, seems to be turning away from fresh healthful foods to frozen and canned goods. No wonder the medical industry is booming.

There is, however, a growing awareness of the value of simple traditional foods for their wonderful taste and health-enhancing properties.

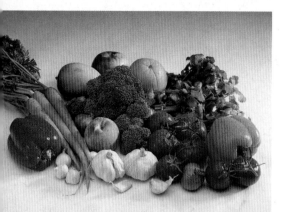

Rediscover the simple remedies and healing agents of raw fruits and vegetabels.

An increasing number of people are realizing that the basis of good health is good nutrition; thus, many people are achieving better health simply by improving their eating habits. It seems that everything else follows.

The first step to improving your diet is to recognize its shortcomings. This is not always easy. The ill effects of the typical North American diet are slow to accumulate and often stay hidden for many years. A high protein intake tends to mask a lack of vitamins, enzymes, minerals and trace elements caused by eating nutrient-deficient vegetables. It may take a while for the toxic by-products produced as a result of metabolizing excess protein to create serious problems. What sometimes develops instead of outright illness is a kind of a twilight condition between health and sickness in which we are well fed, but badly nourished.

The aim of this book is to help those who want to be well nourished. The secret of good nourishment comes mainly from our plant world. Yet fresh vegetables are not always in season so we must look for means of preserving them for use throughout the year. It so happens that there is a method of doing just that—one that has the added benefits of bestowing superior taste and valuable healing properties to vegetables. This method of preservation is lactic acid fermentation.

"Why," you might ask, "should I start preserving my vegetables by fermentation instead of freezing them?" As you will soon learn, lactic acid-fermented vegetables are both great tasting and a component of natural healing. It is time to reacquaint ourselves with the centuries-old technique of lactic acid fermentation. Its methods are simple, but nonetheless they require care and attention for successful results. Getting used to healthier food helps us to strengthen our natural instincts for nutritious eating. Our bodies will learn to recognize what we need. As celebrated German physician, Theophrastus Paracelsus said, "Simplicity is the key."

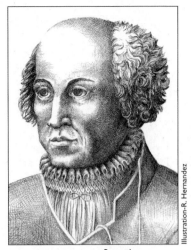

Illustration-R. Hernandez

Paracelsus
1493-1541

All About Kraut . . . .

In case you had any doubts, sauerkraut is not about Germans, though two of us, Klaus and Siegfried, are proud to be Krauts. Kraut is merely the southern German and Austrian word for cabbage. *Sauer*, translated to English, means "sour;" thus, sauerkraut is sour cabbage.

There are very special things about sour cabbage and other lactic acid-fermented vegetables that we will discover together. Their great taste, how to prepare them, how to use them in mouth-watering recipes and, most importantly, why they make us and keep us healthy and rejuvenated.

Lactic acid fermentation allows us to eat fresh, locally grown vegetables, rich in enzymes and vitamin C, even in the middle of winter. Sauerkraut is low in calories, provides good roughage and is easily digested—even by people suffering from diabetes and lactose problems. Finally, it can be easily made at home. Store bought sauerkraut in tins is not raw, it is heated and pasteurized and has lost most vitamin C content and enzymes. Most sauerkraut in glass jars is also pasteurized, unless the label says otherwise

From Cultivation to Preservation

As consumers, we should be more aware of the all-important connection between fertilizers and the cultivation of our food plants. Food production is quite different from other forms of production; you can't ensure high quality by simply selecting what looks to be a good final product.

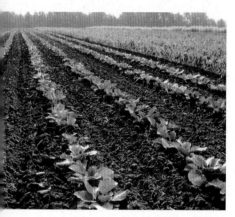

You have to start by ensuring, as far as possible, that the right methods of cultivation have been used. The nutrients in our agricultural lands have been exhausted by over farming and by the use of artificial fertilizers. The soil has been made sterile by chemical herbicides and insecticides and we are left with farmlands that can only produce feeble plants that don't keep well at all. A growing number of consumers are seeking organically grown produce.

Over-farming and the use of artificial fertilizers have exhausted the nutrients in our lands.

The aim of food preservation should be more than to just prevent food from spoiling. Preservation should also add fragrance and aroma and improve digestibility. Lactic acid fermentation, the topic of this book, does all these things. Lactic acid fermentation has played an important role in history because of its health-giving and preservative qualities. Archeological finds have shown that even during the hunter-gatherer stage of human development, people fermented plant food and cabbage.

> ❝ Organically grown cabbage is much easier
> to ferment into sauerkraut than cabbage
> that has been grown in artificially fertilized soil.
> Heavily fertilized cabbage often rots
> before it starts fermenting. ❞

History and Tradition

The Chinese have been fermenting cabbage for thousands of years, and prescribe sauerkraut juice for various physical ailments. One story has it that lactic acid fermentation was discovered accidentally during the building of the Great Wall of China: the poor workers building the wall owned no individual dishes, all foods were dumped into one crock. After a few days, the flavor started changing as the cabbage fermented.

It is recorded as early as 200 BC, that Chinese cooks were pickling cabbage in wine and using it as a condiment.

The first written instructions on lactic acid fermentation are found in the writings of the Roman scholar Pliny in 50 AD. The Romans greatly appreciated sauerkraut and other lactic acid-fermented products. On extended journeys to the Middle East, Emperor Tiberius carried several barrels of sauerkraut as protection against intestinal infections. In medieval Europe, lactic acid-fermented foods were an essential part of the daily meal. But even before that, cabbages were cultivated in ancient Egypt and Greece. In the second century BC, the Greek philosopher Theophrastus mentioned three types of cabbage in his writings on plants. Dioscurides, a Greek physician, wrote of cabbage, "it is healthier if only warmed than cooked." In 200 BC, Cato the Elder praised cabbage as "the very best vegetable."

During the Eastern invasion of Europe, Genghis Khan (1167-1227) carried cabbage fermented with salt, sauerkraut as it is now called, to the eastern edge of Europe. And, as with so many things, the Germans adopted the Slavic method of using lactic acid fermentation and maintained this practice.

China and Japan have used lactic acid fermentation for centuries.

9

Attention was focused on the nutritional importance of sauerkraut when, in the 18th century, sailors often suffered from scurvy, a vitamin C deficiency. Captain Cook sailed around the world, carrying barrels of sauerkraut, not losing a single man to scurvy during his three-year voyage. A new era in navigation began with the introduction of sauerkraut into the seafaring diet.

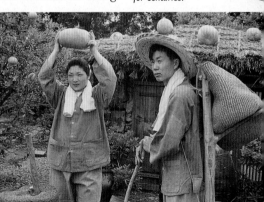

Traditional lactic acid fermentation is of great importance in India and South East Asia, where it is used to preserve fish, fruits and vegetables. There, the technique of preservation is crucial because food spoils rapidly in the warm, moist climate. China and Japan can also boast of age-old methods of lactic acid fermentation. Miso, which gives soup a meaty flavor, is one product that the Japanese ferment from soybeans, rice and barley. Traditionally, the preparation of miso is an annual ritual during which the otherwise hard-to-digest soy protein is refined into a valuable dietary staple.

Eating in Russia and the Balkans is unthinkable without lactic acid-fermented products. There, people have long enjoyed kefir and yogurt, as well as a fermented product common to North Americans, sourdough bread. The Russian national dish, kapusta, is a mixture of white cabbage, tomatoes, carrots, apples, pears, cucumbers and lots of herbs. Borscht, the traditional Russian soup, is made with lactic acid-fermented beets.

**❝In Korea, as well as in parts of Japan,
a meal is not complete without kimchi,
a lactic fermented vegetable.❞**

About Lactic Acid Bacteria

The whitish film on organic fruits and vegetables is beneficial.

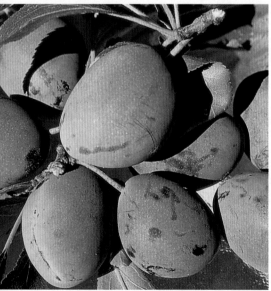

Lactic acid is formed as a product of energy exchange during the metabolism of microorganisms and other life forms, both plants and animals. The name is derived from the Latin word for milk, as the bacteria were first isolated in sour milk. The salts of lactic acid are known as "lactates." Lactic acid bacteria cause catabolic changes in certain sugars. The changes result in two new products: lactic acid and carbon dioxide. The lactic acid breaks down foods, making them more easily digestible. The lactic acid process brings about another boon: the natural preservation of the fermented food. There are, in fact, two kinds of lactic acid bacteria: one that is adapted to milk and milk products, and one that is adapted to plants.

Bacterial floras are responsible for providing lactic acid to the mucous membranes in the mouth, the intestines and the female genital organs. In the plant kingdom, species growing close to the soil have the most lactic acid bacteria. It is important to note that almost all vegetables are plentifully supplied by nature with lactic acid-forming bacteria. Traditional methods of lactic acid fermentation preservation (that do not involve the addition of a bacterial culture to start fermentation) rely strongly on this fact. Vegetables and fruits provide their own lactic acid bacteria. The white film you find on fruits, like plums, apples and grapes is the yeast that starts the fermentation process and turns the fruit sugar into alcohol. The same white film on cabbage and other vegetables is the beneficial bacteria that starts the fermentation process and turns vegetable carbohydrates into lactic acid. Likewise, unpasteurized milk sours by itself. The friendly bacteria from the grass the cow grazed on are carried into the milk and turn the milk sugar (lactose) into lactic acid. Adding a starter culture, like lactobacillus acidophilus bulgaricus, yogurt or kefir, to make sour milk is only necessary with milk that has been pasteurized.

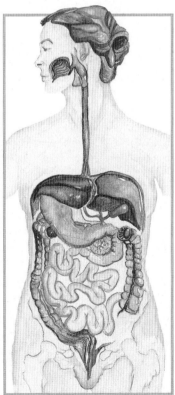

Lactic acid-fermented products are good for the digestive system.

Friendly Bacteria and Health

Lactic acid bacteria prevent decay not only in food products but in the bowels as well. Acetylcholine, which is produced during fermentation, stimulates the peristaltic movement of the intestines. It assists the circulation of the blood and prevents constipation by promoting bowel movements. Lactic acid-fermented products have a harmonizing effect on the stomach: they strengthen the acidity of the gastric juice when hydrochloric acid production lags, and reduce acidity when production is up. Lactic acid acts like a key that fits neatly into the secretion glands of the stomach–to lock and unlock the glands according to the needs of the organism. Lactic acid maintains the balance between acids and alkalis. Lactic acid also encourages the function of the pancreas, which in turn stimulates the secretions of all the digestive organs. Of special importance to people with diabetes is the fact that the carbohydrates in lactic acid-fermented

11

foods have already been broken down and do not, therefore, make heavy demands on the pancreas.

Lactic acid-fermented products are excellent for those with weakened digestive systems, often the result of eating nutritionally poor foods, exposure to pollution and disease.

Lactic acid-fermented food is also a useful addition to the diet of cancer patients, where it serves as an effective supplemental treatment.

"Much doesn't help much" is an old saying that holds true for the use of lactic acid-fermented vegetables. The positive effect of lactic acid-fermented products lies in their regular use, not in consuming vast quantities sporadically. Accordingly, consuming three to four tablespoonfuls of sauerkraut daily, preferably raw, can be sufficient to ward off disease, constipation and other intestinal problems.

Pasteurization

Pasteurization is the process of heating foods such as milk and vegetables to kill any bacteria or microorganisms that could cause disease. In the case of pasteurized vegetables, however, this process also kills off the healthy lactic acid bacteria which aids digestion, fights disease and imparts superior flavours. Most commercially available sauerkraut is pasteurized merely to improve its shelf-life—but be under no illusions, the pasteurized product does not hold the same healing properties that the naturally fermented product does.

What you Need . . . .

Crocks, Pots and Jars

The idea of having a special crock for fermentation is an ancient one. In China and Korea such containers have been used for thousands of years. There are, of course, a variety of containers you can use to pickle vegetables, and as we will see, each has its own advantages and disadvantages.

Open Stoneware Pots

If you prefer to use a traditional open stoneware pot, fill about 75 percent of the pot with crushed vegetables and cover them with a clean linen cloth. Then put a weight stone on top of the cloth. A water and acid-proof stone such as granite must be used—limestone or marble will dissolve in the carbonic acid. If you do not have a suitable stone, put a plate or board on top that covers the vegetables as much as possible. Birch or beech are the woods traditionally used for this purpose. Don't use fir or pine. Their strong odors are easily transferred to the vegetables.

With the traditional kind of fermentation crock, keeping the fermenting vegetables free of kahm yeast can be a real problem. The open pots have to be tended very carefully. The white yeast, or kahm, which develops on the top, must be removed every 10 to 14 days, discarding the top portion of your sauerkraut. At the same time, the cloth, board and stone that cover the vegetables have to be washed or boiled. You can fasten a plastic bag over the pot to protect the contents from air.

Kahm yeast isn't harmful but because it gives the cabbage a bad taste it must be regularly removed. This continuous problem is no doubt one of the reasons why people turned away from lactic acid fermentation to other preservation methods.

Harsch Crock

The good news for sauerkraut lovers is that a new fermentation crock manufactured by Harsch, a German company, has a patented gutter and lid that does away with the need for the constant cleaning. Kept in a cool place, this new crock can be left alone for months while the vegetables inside get better and better. The only maintenance that the new crock requires is that you occasionally top up the water in the gutter that seals the contents from outside air.

Not only the design, but the materials and process used in the manufacture of this stoneware crock are new. Covered with a lead-free glaze, it doesn't easily pick up the flavor of the various vegetables that ferment in it, and it is very easy to clean. The thick sides of this crock make it quite heavy, but its life expectancy is almost limitless. Instead of the weak handle of the traditional pots that tended to break easily, the Harsch crock features sturdy carrying handles that cannot break. In addition to serving as handles, they add to the stability of the gutter by acting as buttresses.

The crock comes with two small, semicircular stoneware "weight stones" that are designed to rest on top of the vegetables to create the pressure necessary for fermentation, and to protect the food from decay. Like the crock itself, the weight stones will not take on the aroma or flavor of the fermenting vegetables.

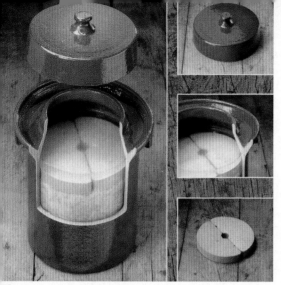

The new Harsch crock has the fermentation lock that guaranties perfect sauerkraut.

With the Harsch crock there is no need for the traditional paraphernalia of cloth, board or stone—and the kahm yeast no longer forms. During fermentation, carbonic acid forms and the water-filled gutter keeps this carbonic acid in the crock where it prevents the formation of kahm yeast. Excess carbon dioxide can, however, escape through the water seal. A happy little "gloop-gloop" noise will let you know when this is happening.

The carbonic acid layer that accumulates in the crock combines with free oxygen and water. This process creates a vacuum that should not be disturbed.

When adding ingredients, take care to allow space for the accumulating carbonic acid by leaving at least an inch (2.5 cm) of free space at the top. There should be at least an inch of fluid or brine covering the weight stones. If the fluid level drops below the stones, top it up with boiled salted water (use a ratio of one tablespoon of salt to one quart or litre of water). Do not be alarmed if suddenly all the water seems to disappear from the gutter; just move the lid slightly (don't lift it!) and you will notice that the water is still there—the vacuum has merely drawn it upward inside the lid.

After emptying, it is easy to clean the glazed fermentation crock as well as the lid and the weight stones. All the different parts must be cleaned thoroughly.

Preserving Jars

You can use ordinary glass preserving jars for fermentation if you wish, or any glass jar with a twist lid. The essential thing is that the lids close tightly. Check the lids of used vacuum jars carefully as they may have been damaged when the jar was opened. You might have to use double rubber rings to get a good, tight seal if you are using preserving jars. Prepare the food in the same way as you would if you were using a fermentation crock. You can then press the vegetables into the jar, making sure you don't fill it to more than 80 percent of its capacity.

When preserving in jars there should always be one-half inch (1 cm) of brine on top of all fermenting vegetables as some liquid will escape the jar as vapor. The sealed jars should also be stored on a towel, as any escaping liquid will dribble down the sides.

The jars must be kept in the dark during the fermentation stage and subsequent storage. Put them in a carton, or cover them with a cloth. Using smaller containers like twist-top jars can be more practical for small families and single people. It is, however, easier to obtain good results when working with larger amounts of vegetables because a larger number of microorganisms will then be interacting with each other. Plastic jars are not recommended as harmful substances can leech into preserved foods over time.

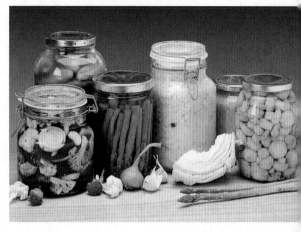

Preserving jars must be kept in the dark during fermentation.

Utensils

No matter what containers you use, it is imperative that they are squeaky clean. Use hot water on the pots and avoid strong detergents. Let the pots dry in the open air or in the sun, if possible. Shredding is often necessary in lactic acid-fermented preserves. Crushing is a good alternative, and you will sometimes want to do both. Use your discretion. If you expect to be preparing large quantities of vegetables for lactic acid fermentation, invest in a large wooden crusher or potato masher for pressing the vegetables tightly into the jars, and a whetstone to sharpen your knives for shredding.

Vegetables Recommended for Fermentation

Beans	Celery	Peppers
Beets	Cucumbers	Rutabagas
Cabbage (White, Red, Savoy)	Kohlrabi	Tomatoes
Cauliflower	Leaks	Turnips
	Onions	

Picking the Best Vegetables

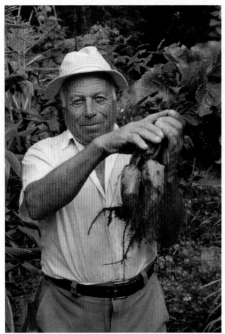

If you are a gardener, you get to choose when your vegetables are harvested. There are, however, some minor rules to obey. For instance, don't harvest vegetables destined for preservation directly after a rainy period. Wait a day or two. Lactic acid bacteria are present on most plants as surface culture, and their numbers diminish during rainy weather. If you're the gardener you can also avoid the use of pesticides or artificial fertilizers, which will wreak havoc with the original flora. Hopefully, your soil will be rich in nutrients. Lactic acid bacteria are very demanding about their nourishment; they need fermentable sugar, minerals, trace elements and almost all the B vitamins for their development.

Don't use pesticides or artificial fertilizers in our garden.

Clean the vegetables well, making sure they are free of soil. An interesting way of preserving, and one that is still common in Romania and Bulgaria, is to leave the vegetables whole.

We have always had good results with preserving whole vegetables. In a cool, dark basement, lactic acid-fermented vegetables will keep for a year or more.

Beans

Beans are the only vegetables that have to be cooked before preservation. They contain a toxic substance called phasin, a protein that interferes with digestion and decomposes when heated. Never serve raw beans on a salad plate!

Cut, wax and string beans, as well as broad or "tick" beans are suitable for lactic acid fermentation. The more tender the beans, the better the end result. Be careful not to over-salt your beans.

beans

Basic Lactic Acid-Fermented Beans

(for a one quart/litre preserving jar)

> **3 ½ cups beans**
> **½ small onion**
> **savory**
> **3 tbsp pickling or sea salt**
> **2 tbsp whey**

Boil beans in lightly salted water (2 tbsp pickling or sea salt to 1 quart/litre of water) for five to ten minutes. For very tender beans, five minutes cooking time is enough. For larger amounts, cook one batch after the other in the same water. Take care in all cases to avoid overcooking. Spread them on a cloth to cool. Next, layer the beans in the preserving jar together with the savory and onion. Mix the whey with the water in which you boiled the beans, and pour this mixture so that there is ½ inch (1 cm) of liquid on top of the vegetables.

Leave the container at room temperature (64-68°F or 18-20°C), for eight to ten days, then put it in a cool place. After three weeks of storage the beans will be ready for consumption.

Beans with Mustard and Dill

Follow recipe above, adding 1 tsp yellow mustard seeds, 1 tbsp freshly-grated horseradish, 1 clove of garlic, savory and dill blossoms to the jar.

Beets

Beets have been used for medicinal purposes for two thousand years. Their rich chemical and mineral composition gives them a wide range of medicinal functions. It has now been scientifically shown that the beet promotes cell respiration and stimulates the immune system. This promotes the recovery and normalization of tissues that have already begun to develop toward cancer.

Having said this, it is not all that easy to ferment beets. Your best bet is to preserve them together with white cabbage, onions and apples. If you do beets alone they will produce a thick, slimy juice that, although very aromatic and tasty, does not keep well. If you are going to preserve them alone, don't do too many at one time.

Lactic Acid-Fermented Beets

(for a one quart/litre preserving jar)

> **3½ cups beets, peeled and chopped**
> **1 tsp mustard seeds**
> **¼ tsp caraway seeds**
> **1 tbsp horseradish, chopped** (available at farmer's or
>   Chinese markets)
> **¼ cup onions, coarsely chopped**
> **boiled salt water for filling up the container**
>   (1½ tbsp salt to 1 quart/litre water)
> **1 tsp whey** (see page 28)
> **lactic acid-fermented juice** (optional)

Layer the beets in the jar with the onions, mustard, caraway seeds and horseradish, filling the jar only three-quarters full, as beets ferment heavily. Add boiled salt water, whey and lactic acid-fermented juice until they are just covered. Leave the pot at room temperature (64-68°F or 20-24°C) for two to three days. Then store at a temperature of 64°F (18°C) for no longer than ten days. Finally, store in a cool place.

White Cabbage

The synthesis for protein, carbohydrates and fats takes place in cabbage leaves.

Cabbage originated in Europe. Throughout the history of human nutrition, white cabbage and its relatives have played an important role. The great American biochemist Ebert McCollum points out that the leaf of this plant is a complete food in itself.

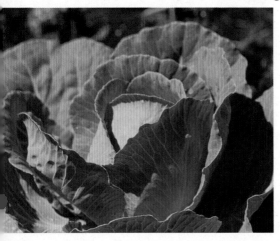

Researcher Hans Rudolf Locher confirms that every form of cabbage has healing powers. He states that the juiciest, darkest and greenest leaves are the most effective for external applications in cases such as abscesses, bronchial asthma, bronchitis, pleurisy, gangrene, gout, bruises, contusions, crush injuries, and inflammations of the lymph nodes and the middle ear. In all of these conditions, the external and internal use of sauerkraut brings about healing.

The synthesis of protein, carbohydrates and fats takes place in cabbage leaves. The active cells that perform these tasks contain everything that is essential for our metabolism. This vegetable is so rich in nutrients and lactic acid bacteria that it can normally be relied on to start and sustain its own lactic acid fermentation process with no trouble at all.

Sauerkraut made from summer cabbage is ready for consumption after only fourteen days. It is delicious but not too durable. You should only ferment as much as you can eat within a fairly short time. For winter consumption, autumn cabbage is best. The essential point is to use only mature, sound cabbage.

Simple Sauerkraut

(for a seven quart/litre fermentation pot)

> **12 lbs** (6 kg) **white cabbage**
> **½ tbsp caraway seeds**
> **3 sour apples** (optional)
> **4 tbsp pickling or sea salt**

Low-Salt Sauerkraut

(for a seven quart/litre fermentation pot)

> **12 lbs** (6 kg) **white cabbage**
> **1 ½ cups chopped onions**
> **½ tbsp caraway seeds**
> **6 juniper berries**
> **1½ tbsp pickling or sea salt**
> **1 quart/litre whey** (see page 28)

Salt-Free Sauerkraut

(for a seven quart/litre fermentation pot)

> **12 lbs** (6 kg) **white cabbage**
> **1 quart/litre whey**
> **juice of 2 lemons**
> **2 oz** (50 g) **glucose** (in health food stores)

The vitamin C content is highest in the green leaves, so don't imagine that the snow-white specimens are necessarily the best cabbages. Some of the outermost green leaves should, however, be removed. You can use them in soups or stews. Remember to save a few big leaves for the final layer. Clean the cabbage, cut out any bruised sections and the stalk-which should not be thrown away. It contains fermentable sugar and fine aromatic substances. Shred it on a coarse grater and mix it in with the cut and crushed leaves of the cabbage.

Mix all ingredients in a large bowl. Transfer this mix to the crock or preservation jar a bit at a time and pack the mix tightly. Repeat this process until the pot is about 80 percent full. Cover the last layer with a few large leaves. Do not over fill, as fermentation will expand the cabbage, and you have to leave room for the weight stones. The water must cover the weight stones while still leaving a one inch (2.5 cm) of air space at the top. If you are using a Harsch crock, put the lid on the fermentation pot and fill up the gutter with water.

Put the pot in a warm place. The temperature should be between 68° and 72°F (20-22°C) for a few days. After fermentation has started, put the pot in a cool place for two to three weeks. In order for a slow fermentation to take place the temperature should be around 59°F (15°C).

Only after this time should you open the pot. You might have to rinse the stones and pour boiled, cooled salted water over the cabbage if it has dried. After that, put the pot in a cold place, ideally between 32° and 50°F (0-10°C). You can eat the sauerkraut after four weeks, but it will be even better if you leave it for a longer period.

Red Cabbage

Red cabbage can be preserved in the same way as white cabbage. However, red cabbage, has to be pressed thoroughly with a potato masher, as it is a very hard vegetable, until enough juice is extracted to cover the kraut. Fill up the fermentation pot with a bit of whey or some lactic acid-fermented vegetable juice from sauerkraut or fermented cucumbers.

Lactic Acid-Fermented Red Cabbage

(for a seven quart/litre fermentation pot)

12 lbs. (6 kg.) **red cabbage**
3 sour apples
2 medium sized onions
2-4 bay leaves
¼ tsp caraway seeds
6-8 juniper berries
4 tbsp pickling or sea salt
¼ quart/litre whey (optional)

Preparation is the same as for white cabbage sauerkraut.

❝Cabbage could be in medical science what bread is in nutrition; cabbage is the physician of the poor.❞

Dr. Blanc, Parisian physician, 1881

Celery Root

Celery roots contain a whole bouquet of aromatic scents and are therefore well suited for mixing with milder kinds of vegetables. There is hardly a combination in which you will not appreciate its rich flavor. You will also get good results if you preserve celery roots with only onions and herbs.

Select medium-sized, hard cucumbers for fermentation.

Cucumbers

Fresh, lactic acid-fermented cucumbers with their mild acidity and spicy taste are universal favorites.

Cucumbers grow rapidly during warm, humid summers. In conditions such as these, they also ferment rapidly. If, on the other hand, the summer has been cold and dry, it is important to add whey and a little more salt to prevent the cucumbers from turning soft. In Finland and Russia, during cool summers in which fermentation is slower, housewives put a few oak leaves into the fermentation container. The tannic

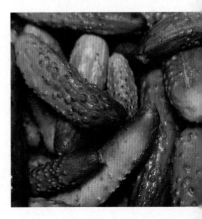

acid of the oak helps to protect the cucumbers from decomposition until enough lactic acid has formed.

Select medium-sized, hard cucumbers for fermentation. Clean and brush them to rid them of any dirt. Poke holes into them with a knitting needle or a sharp knife to facilitate the exchange of fluids. Larger cucumbers have to be cut into pieces.

Lactic Acid-Fermented Cucumbers

(for a one quart/litre preserving jar)

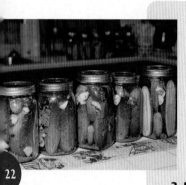

3 cups cucumbers
I bay leaf
½ tsp pickling or sea salt
½ small onion, sliced in rings or quartered
I clove garlic, finely chopped
I tbsp fresh horseradish root, chopped
     (available in farmer's or Chinese markets)
I tsp mustard seeds
lots of fresh dill
I stem fresh tarragon
3-5 ground coriander seeds
boiled salt water for filling up the container
    (I¼ tbsp salt to I quart/litre water)
I tbsp wine vinegar (optional)

Horseradish keeps pickled cucumbers crisp for a long time, 'knackig' as the Germans say.

Pack the cucumbers, onion, garlic, tomato, horseradish and herbs firmly into the preserving jar until the container is 80 percent full. Fill the jar with salted water, making sure there is a ½ inch (1 cm) layer of liquid on top of the cucumbers and seal tight. Leave the container at room temperature for ten days, then put it in a cold place. Cucumbers will be ready to eat after two to three weeks of cold storage.

Lactic acid-fermented cucumbers go well with bread and in salads. You can also make a sandwich spread or sauce from lactic acid-fermented cucumbers and onions. Simply mince the cucumbers and onions and add parsley and chives. Mix with some mustard and curds or sour cream.

Pumpkin and Squash

A few years ago, when calories were the be-all and end-all of dieting, the fortunes of pumpkins went into decline. But now we have begun to realize that excessive protein and refined foods also play a part in weight gain. Proper nutrition is an important component in weight control and this traditional stand-by, with its marvelous cleansing and detoxifying qualities, is coming into its own once again.

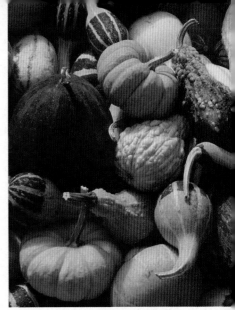

Pumpkins chosen for lactic acid fermentation should not be too ripe or they will fall apart during fermentation. If they do fall apart, you needn't follow suit! Your lactic acid-fermented pumpkin will still be tasty and nutritious, even if it is a little hard to handle.

Pumpkin and Squash have cleansing and detoxifying qualities.

As pumpkin lacks a strong taste of its own, you can add plenty of spices to make sure that the end product doesn't turn out too bland.

Lactic Acid-Fermented Pumpkin with Peppers

(for a one quart/litre preserving jar)

2¼ cups pumpkin or squash, peeled and cubed
¼ cup sour apples, chopped but not peeled
⅓ cup green or red peppers, chopped into half-inch squares, seeds and white part removed
4 tbsp minced onions
I clove garlic
¼ tsp whole cloves
2 bay leaves
I tsp mustard seeds
horseradish to taste
I tbsp pickling or sea salt
(If you want to do a really special job, boil the pumpkin peels and the pepper seeds for half an hour and use that water for filling up the preserving jar.)
4 tbsp whey or, lactic acid-fermented juice (optional)

Lactic Acid-Fermented Pumpkin with Lemons and Spice

(for a one quart/litre preserving jar)

3 cups pumpkin or squash
½ lemon, peeled and cubed
¾ cup sour apples chopped but not peeled,
I inch (2 cm) piece fresh ginger root, chopped
4-5 whole cloves
pinch of cinnamon
I tbsp pickling or sea salt
3/4 cup whey, or lactic acid- fermented juice (optional)

Pack layers of fruits and vegetables, herbs and salt very firmly into the jar. Mix whey or lactic acid-fermented juice with the pumpkin/pepper seed stock, or boiled water, and pour this mixture over the vegetables. Pumpkin absorbs water so allow for this by adding a little less water to the jar.

Leave the sealed jar for eight to ten days at a temperature of 64-68°F (18-20°C), then put in cool storage.

Pumpkins can be tailored to suit a wide variety of tastes. Experiment to discover your own favourite flavor combinations!

Pumpkin or Squash Salad Dressing

Lactic acid-fermented pumpkin can be used to supplement all kinds of dishes. It can be puréed in the blender and then used for salad dressings. Add some ground ginger, perhaps some freshly chopped herbs, and a bit of honey. Serve in small bowls as a dip.

Root Vegetables

Root vegetables, in addition to being well-suited to lactic acid fermentation, are potent antioxidants, vitamin-rich and full of fibers that control blood cholesterol levels. The orange-yellow colored vegetables such as carrots and yams are naturally sweet and are excellent sources of beta-carotene–a vitamin essential for the prevention of night-blindness. Root vegetables have the added bonus that they do not spoil quickly, but they do need to be cleaned thoroughly before use.

Basic Recipe for Lactic Acid-Fermented Root Vegetables

(carrots are used in this recipe for a one quart/litre preserving jar)

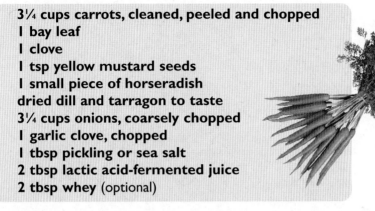

3¼ cups carrots, cleaned, peeled and chopped
1 bay leaf
1 clove
1 tsp yellow mustard seeds
1 small piece of horseradish
dried dill and tarragon to taste
3¼ cups onions, coarsely chopped
1 garlic clove, chopped
1 tbsp pickling or sea salt
2 tbsp lactic acid-fermented juice
2 tbsp whey (optional)

Mix the carrots with salt, herbs and spices. Layer the spiced carrots tightly in the jar with the onions and garlic. Be careful not to mash the vegetables. In case the carrots do not produce enough of their own juice (which will most often be the case), add boiled salt water (2 tbsp of pickling or sea salt to 1 quart/litre of water) until they are just covered so the carrots will absorb more fluid. Leave the pot at room temperature (64-68°F or 18-20°C) for two to three days. Then store at a temperature of 64°F (18°C) for no longer than ten days. Finally, store in a cool place. Root vegetables need at least four to six weeks of fermentation before they are ready to eat.

This root vegetable recipe is very flexible and lends itself to experimentation. You could try, for instance, substituting turnips for half of the carrots in the above recipe. Turnips will produce a mild acidity and impart a very appealing color.

Lactic Acid-Fermented Carrots and Onions

Mixed together, these vegetables make a simple, delicious salad. Onions can be cut in thin rings and eaten as snacks. They are easily digested and go well with all kinds of spreads. Also mix with endives or chicory.

Whole Vegetables

All vegetables can be preserved whole—all you need are big enough containers. In general, you will get a better result if you mix your vegetables rather than preserving one kind at a time. The reason for this is that the nutritional demands of the lactic acid bacteria are met particularly well by the broad spectrum of nutrients found in a variety of different vegetables.

Added Flavors

The following herbs, spices and vegetables are frequently used to enhance flavor in lactic acid fermentation:

Bay leaves	Garlic	Summer Savory
Caraway Seeds	Horseradish	Red Pepper
Cloves	Juniper Berries	Tarragon
Coriander	Onions	Tomatoes
Dill	Pimentos	Yellow Mustard Seeds
	Raspberry Leaves	

Herbs and Spices

It is hard to think of preserving vegetables without using herbs. Can you imagine a pickle without the dill? Sauerkraut without juniper berries and caraway seeds is equally unthinkable.

Herbs are not just used for their wonderful flavors. They are also rich in minerals and trace elements—the very substances that are all too often lacking in our diets. Herbs have another function that is particularly important in preservation: many of them have the ability to prevent decay. Juniper, garlic and horseradish, to mention but a few, have long been used for this purpose, though they are generally more appreciated for their flavors.

Coriander

Coriander is related to dill and caraway and belongs to the "umbelliferous" family, which includes parsley and carrots. Freshly chopped, it has a wonderful aroma—like a mixture of caraway, aniseed and lemon. Use it uncut for preserving.

Garlic

Lactic acid fermentation allows the garlic lover to indulge his or her fancy without jeopardizing social graces. Garlic tastes almost nutty after fermentation, and its hot quality adds a very special flavor to vegetables.

Onions

Don't hold back on the onions when you preserve. They are good for you and for the fermentation process. Lactic acid-fermented onions are also more easily digested, even for people who cannot eat them raw or boiled. Lactic acid fermentation converts the aggressive onion into a mild and pleasant vegetable.

Onions, either whole or cut into a few big chunks, are put directly into the fermentation container and covered with liquid. Be careful though, they can lose their delicious oils very easily if you cut them open and then leave them lying on the kitchen counter.

Raspberry Leaves

Fresh raspberry leaves, as well as black currant leaves, are rich in lactic acid bacteria and also add a delicious flavor to preserves.

Subtle Herbs

Go easy on the pimento and the cloves! You don't want more than a hint of their presence in the preserve, as they can be quite obtrusive in larger amounts. If you still have dill, tarragon and summer savory by the time fall comes around, cut and dry them. They will be useful later on for the preservation of root vegetables.

Tomatoes

Tomatoes, while not herbs, are a valuable supplement in preserves as nourishment for the lactic acid bacteria.

Other Ingredients

Salt

Because many of us are limiting our salt-intake, it's natural that we should question the role of salt in lactic acid fermentation. Vegetables contain proteins in addition to carbohydrates, and proteins tend to spoil when they break down. Salt is used to prevent this from happening, and is especially important in the early stages before the lactic acid has accumulated in sufficient quantities to have a preservative effect. Experience has shown that adding salt that weighs between 0.8 and 1.5 percent of the total weight of the vegetables will result in a product that is both tasty and long-lived. There is absolutely no reason to worry about the small amount of salt used in the fermentation process.

Salt to Cabbage Ratio

- 1 tsp salt to 1 lb (454 g) cabbage
- 4 tbsp salt to 12 lbs (6 kg) cabbage
- 1 tbsp salt to 5 quarts cabbage
- (25 ml salt to 5 litres cabbage) (to be adjusted)

Use only Rock salt (real salt), pickling salt or sea salt (Celtic salt), never iodized table salt. Sea salt is excellent for lactic acid fermentation because it contains many minerals and trace elements.

If there is not enough salt, the yeast takes over, which brings about decay. If this is your first try at fermenting vegetables, stick to the recommended amount of salt until you are more experienced. Using the Harsch fermentation crock will minimize the need for salt. Vegetables grown organically require less salt because of their superior quality. And cabbage is the only vegetable that can be fermented with very little salt or no salt at all–most likely because its leaves are particularly rich in vitamins, minerals and naturally-occurring lactic acid.

Water

Unlike spring water, tap water containing chlorine must be boiled, to evaporate the chlorine. As mentioned, you have to add salt to any water you put into the crock. Without salt fermentation will not start. Always boil water, and add the salt while the water is still hot, making sure the salt completely dissolves.

Whey

To make your own whey, line a strainer with a thin cloth and pour some warmed buttermilk, kefir or sour milk into it. The fluid that strains through is whey. Because it contains lactose and several vitamins and minerals, whey is an excellent aid to start the fermentation process. It is essential to add whey to all vegetables, except cabbage and cucumbers, which without help will start fermenting very slowly or may not ferment at all.

A pint or one-half litre of sour milk, buttermilk or kefir yields one-half pint or one-quarter litre of whey. If you have access to fresh cows' milk you can strain your whey from milk that has not been pasteurized. When placed in a warm spot, it will sour within a day or two. This will give you the best and most natural whey. Don't throw away the curds (quark) left behind in the strainer, as they are delicious by themselves or in any number of recipes.

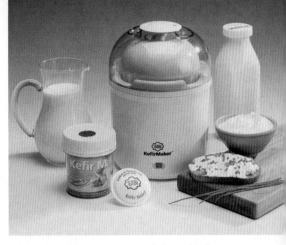

Fermented milk products, such as kefir, are healthy choices

Starter Cultures

We are often asked if there is a reliable starting culture that can be used to get the lactic acid fermentation process off to a good start. You can use juice from a previous lactic acid-fermented preserve, but this really doesn't guarantee success. As we have said, lactic acid fermentation is a dynamic process, and the bacterial composition of the finished product is very different from that found in the first stages of lactic acid fermentation. So, if you use high quality, fresh vegetables, add the right herbs, and follow instructions, you shouldn't have any problems getting the lactic acid fermentation process off to a fine start. Remember: organically grown vegetables come with their own "indigenous" lactic acid fermentation bacteria.

Do use a starting culture, though, if you wish. A lot of the best lactic acid fermentation information will come out of your own experience.

Some vegetables, like cucumbers, produce plenty of juice during fermentation that can be used as a starter culture. Strain off this juice and store it in clean, dark bottles. There must be no air space left in the bottles. If you seal them properly, the contents will keep for ages. Discard the white shell that may form over the contents: it is the same harmless kahm yeast that we spoke about earlier. This juice can be used as a starting culture, or as a dressing instead of vinegar, or as an aperitif before meals. Besides lactic acid, this juice contains minerals, vitamins and acetylcholine.

66Cabbage is the physician of the poor.99

Parisian physician, Dr. Blanc (1881)

The Science of Successful Lactic Acid Fermentation

The art of successful lactic acid fermentation consists of creating four conditions; otherwise the food doesn't ferment, it spoils.

Lactic acid fermentation has four basic requirements:
- a certain concentration of salt
- a specific temperature
- an oxygen-free environment
- pressure on the foods being fermented

Step 1
Grate cabbage into a large bowl

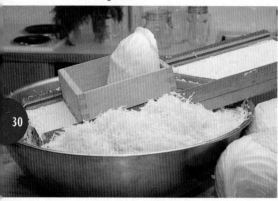

A special kind of fermentation occurs during which lactic acid is formed. Microorganisms, yeast and bacteria all play a role in this process. These organisms can only develop, however, if suitable conditions prevail and if they receive enough nourishment.

The process of lactic acid fermentation occurs in two different phases. First, there is a slight decomposition due to fermentation. The salt initially protects all vegetables from decay until enough lactic acid has formed. Eventually so much acid is produced that the bacteria that cause decay and the butyric acid (a fatty acid that inhibits the fermentation process) can no longer be produced. Yeast fungi, which contribute to the delicious and characteristic fermentation aroma, are also part of the initial fermentation process.

Step 2
Add salt and spices

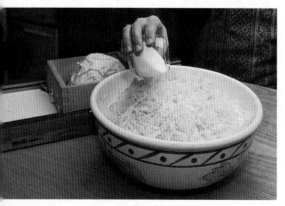

A successful first phase is the foundation on which the whole lactic acid fermentation process rests. It must take place quickly and must not be interrupted. In this first phase, temperature plays an important role. The ideal temperature for sauerkraut is 20-22°C (68-72°F); for cucumbers 18-20°C (64-68°F); and for carrots around 20°C (68°F).

After two days another phase begins: the lactic acid-producing

30

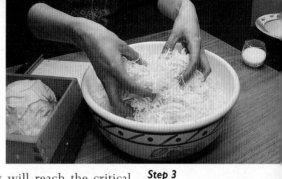

bacteria start gaining the upper hand and eliminate all other bacteria. This process must not be rushed. Lower the temperature to 59-64°F (15-18°C) for cabbage and to about 18°C (64°F) for other vegetables. Fermentation should continue without any problem. Soon, it will reach the critical pH of 4.1, where butyric acid and decay bacteria can no longer form. It is during this phase that new substances like acetylcholine, vitamin C, vitamin B12 and enzymes are formed.

Step 3
Mix together the cabbage and spices

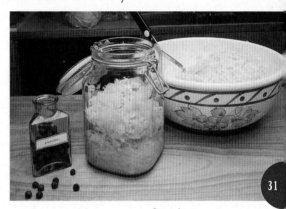

When fermentation stops–after 10 to 14 days (two to three weeks for cabbage)–the vegetables must be put in a cool place, ideally between 8-10°C (46-50°F). A thermometer set on top of the fermentation crock will show whether the temperature is right.

It is important not to open the fermentation crock before the end of fermentation; if you do, the carbon dioxide that prevents yeast formation will escape. If you are using a Harsch crock, check occasionally to ensure that the water gutter is filled. If you use jars with twist lids, put them in a cool place 45-50 F (8-10 C) for ten days without opening them. If you use open containers, the kahm layer must be removed in the way described in the section on open stoneware pots (page 13).

31

Step 4
Add juniper berries where indicated

Step 5
Using a pototo masher, pack the cabbage mix tightly into the jar, one layer at a time while juice builds up on the surface.

Once the vegetables have been put in a cool place, patience is required, as all biological processes need time. Acid formation only takes place during the first, or warm, stage. (It is better, by the way, to make the warm period a little too long rather than too short.) Aroma develops during the cool storage period. To develop the aroma, bacteria need sugar and other nutrients. If all the sugar present has been used up during an overly long and warm fermentation, your product will be well

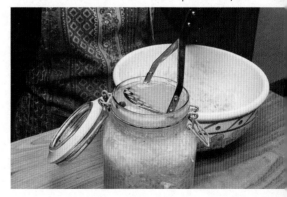

preserved, but it will taste sour, so, stick to suggested fermentation times.

Has the Fermentation Been Successful?

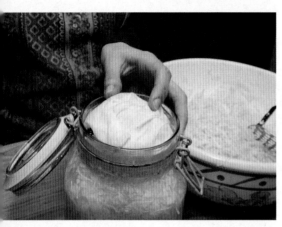

The aroma and taste of your product will tell you. A successful fermentation develops a characteristic, pleasing aroma. The taste should be pleasant and slightly sour. If you do not want to rely on your tongue alone, buy some litmus paper at your local drugstore and test the pH-value.

We should briefly explain that pH-value is a measure of the degree of acidity or alkalinity of a fluid, and is rated on a scale of one to fourteen. The lower the pH, the more acidic the fluid.

Step 6-7
Place a cabbage leaf on top, press firmly down so that brine covers the leaf. Seal the container

Around the middle, at pH 7, the solution is neutral. Above pH 7, the solution is alkaline. For lactic acid fermentation, the critical pH is 4.1. Below this value, decay cannot occur. Decomposition or decay has its own characteristic and unpleasant smell; when this happens, butyric acid forms, and the vegetables turn slimy. Throw them away and try again!

Common Problems

■ Vegetables grown too rapidly, or those over-fertilized or sprayed with pesticides can spoil during fermentation.
■ The water level on top of Harsch crock dried out permitting oxygen to enter the fermentation pot.
■ The pickling jars did not close properly (check seals carefully), permitting oxygen to enter jars.
■ Fermentation can also fail if insufficient salt was used. Salt is the preservative to bridge the time until lactic acid is formed.

Storing Your Lactic Acid-Fermented Vegetables

It is important that you do not open the fermentation crock too often. Calculate your needs for two or three weeks, remove that quantity from the fermentation crock, transfer it into twist top jars and put them in the fridge. Open jars of lactic acid-fermented vegetables must be kept cool. If you wish, you can pour cold-pressed oil on top of the contents to minimize their exposure to air.

When you have used up two-thirds of the vegetables in the fermentation crock, transfer the remainder into smaller jars in order to free up the big one for further use.

Healing With Lactic Acid Fermentation . . . . .

66It is truly a broom for the stomach and intestines. It takes away the bad juices and gases, strengthens the nerves and stimulates blood formation. You should eat it even if other cabbage is forbidden in your diet. Eat it moderately, well-chewed, and do not drink anything with it. 99

Father Kneipp, 19th century natural healer

Medicine from the Kitchen

Hippocrates, the father of medicine, demanded that our nourishment be curative, and that our cures be nourishing. In modern times, his words still have urgency and significance.

Lactic acid-fermented vegetables supremely fulfill Hippocrates' ideal of nutritious and curative nourishment. They are not only tasty, but they also exert stimulating and healing effects.

Modern research confirms what people have long known from experience. Lactic acid bacteria create an environment in the intestines in which harmful bacteria that are sensitive to acidity, such as those causing cholera and typhoid, just cannot develop. Our bodies work in symbiosis with intestinal flora. Sauerkraut eliminates disease-causing bacteria and reintroduces friendly bacteria (such as Lactobacillus acidophilus). Such friendly bacteria, which are often destroyed by antibiotic residues in our

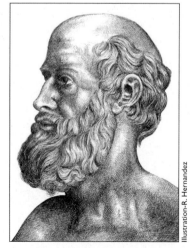

Hippocrates
460-375 BC

Illustration-R. Hernandez

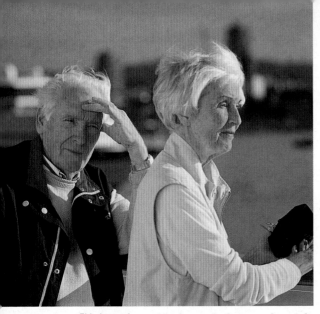

food, are necessary for healthy digestion and proper elimination of waste products.

In the process of fermentation, the carbohydrates in the vegetables break down and form lactic acid, which activates the gastric juices and thus helps to break down the ingested food for correct assimilation. Since lactic acid is a strong acid, it can in part replace the hydrochloric acid present in the stomach. This is of particular benefit to the elderly and those who otherwise experience a weakness of hydrochloric acid and other enzyme production. With age, the digestive organs weaken. While raw foods are often not well tolerated by the elderly, lactic acid-fermented vegetables are already broken down by the fermentation process and are, therefore, easily digestible.

Elderly people often experience a weakness of hydrocloric acid and other enzyme production.

Lactic acid fermentation is a good method of preserving vegetables, and eating vegetables preserved in this way is an effective way to attain health and maintain it. Our body certainly does not need huge amounts of lactic acid-fermented vegetables—we don't have to eat sauerkraut until we are stuffed! Small amounts, taken regularly, are quite sufficient to initiate many healing processes.

Nutrients in Sauerkraut

Lactic acid-fermented vegetables—and sauerkraut in particular—are highly nutritious and low in calories. They also contain high amounts of vitamins and minerals. A half-cup portion of sauerkraut contains the following nutrients:

- 20 calories (kcal)
- 1.1 g protein
- 0.2 g fat
- 3.4 g carbohydrate
- 1.4 g raw fiber
- traces of vitamin A
- 20 mcg vitamin B1

- 200 mcg vitamin B2
- 18 mg vitamin C
- 730 mg sodium
- 490 mg potassium
- 31 mg phosphorus
- 46 mg calcium
- 0.5 mg iron

Lactose Intolerance

Lactic acid-fermented foods are well-tolerated by people who have problems digesting lactose. In the human intestines, lactose is split into its components of glucose and galactose through the action of the enzyme lactase, before entering the bloodstream. Additionally, small quantities of lactose reach the lower intestines and are converted into lactic acid by the intestinal flora. For this reason, lactose has a positive effect on the intestinal flora and the general condition of the lower bowels. The toning action of lactose is important for rebuilding the intestinal flora following antibiotic treatment, or in the case of chronic constipation.

Some lactose intolerance is caused by a deficiency in the enzyme lactase. Lactose intolerance can also be the result of a digestive tract disease. Older people can become somewhat more lactose intolerant than they were in their younger years, when there were still sufficient amounts of lactase generated in their systems.

When lactose is incompletely digested, larger than normal amounts reach the lower bowels where they are fermented by intestinal bacteria. This can give rise to bloating, diarrhea and cramping. Fortunately, lactose intolerant people can still enjoy lactic acid-fermented foods like sauerkraut because fermented lactose is more easily digested by the lower bowels than regular lactose.

Boosting the Metabolism with Enzymes

Lactic acid-fermented vegetables activate the pancreas causing the level of sugar in the blood and the urine to lessen (good news for people with diabetes!). Since the vegetables (with the exception of green beans) are not heated during the fermentation process, their enzymes, which are susceptible to chemicals as well as to heat, are preserved. Enzymes play a crucial role in our metabolism; without them, metabolic activity would be extraordinarily slow.

Lowering Blood Pressure

Eating sauerkraut (and lactic acid-fermented vegetables in general) lowers of blood pressure. This hypotensive effect is based on sauerkraut's choline content. Choline is a substance that balances and regulates the composition of the blood. On top of that, choline also lowers the level of fats in the blood.

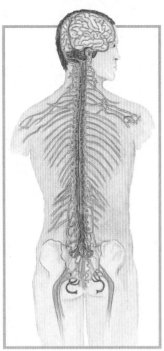

Acetylchlorine has a calming effect on the nervous system.

Calming the Nervous System

Another vital substance present in sauerkraut, is acetylcholine, a compound released at many autonomic nerve endings, and believed to have a specific function in the transmission of nerve impulses. Acetylcholine has a pronounced calming effect on the nervous system and, as mentioned earlier, stimulates the peristaltic movement of the intestines. It also improves sleep patterns, lowers blood pressure and strengthens the heart. However, acetylcholine is susceptible to heat. This means that in order to get the full therapeutic effect, sauerkraut should not be cooked.

Holistic Cancer Therapy

Lactic acid-fermented vegetables are firmly established as healing agents in holistic cancer therapies. In his book *Internal Cancer Therapy and the Nutrition of the Cancer Patient*, Dr. Werner Zabel draws attention to the fact that the presence of a cancerous growth is always accompanied by a lack of hydrochloric acid and of enzymes. Regular consumption of lactic acid-fermented foods, especially sauerkraut, provides the body with the necessary hydrochloric acid and enzymes. If our food is poorly digested and decomposed, our intestines become overloaded with metabolic toxins that must then be processed by the liver.

Most modern guides to natural healing methods recommend regular intake of lactic acid as co-therapy for cancer. Many cancer researchers, among them Kuhl, Scheller, Kleine, Herberger and Zabel, advocate holistic approaches to cancer that focus on lactic acid fermented food sources such as sauerkraut. Today it is well known that cancer is rampant in countries where food intake is highly processed, and rare in countries where diets consist mainly of fresh or lactic acid fermented foods.

It is clear that in cancer cases, food consumption should consist of more lactic acid-fermented foods (vegetables and milk products) because the lactic acid helps the intestinal flora that is often impaired by cancers. Lactic acid helps to produce B-vitamins via the intestinal flora. It also stimulates cell metabolism, which is severely impaired by cancer. Lactic acid also detoxifies. Lactic acid-fermented vegetables, provided they are made with high-quality raw materials (i.e., organic cabbage, raw certified milk, etc.), are effective in helping normalize cell respiration, metabolism and the crucial acid-alkaline or pH-balance of the body.

According to cancer researcher Kleine, and following the research of O. Th. Weiss, patients with intestinal cancer should avoid fermented milk products and instead use lactic acid-fermented vegetable products, as the vegetable-derived lactic acid fermentation is more effective with this particular type of cancer. The special medicinal importance of lactic acid-fermented vegetables and their juices, and in particular sauerkraut, is thoroughly investigated and addressed in various books by Dr. Johannes Kuhl, including *Checkmate to Cancer*.

Kuhl states that "lactic acid is the functional element of growth in nature and the regenerative component for damaged plant and animal cells. The lactic acid-containing products, like no other nutrients, have an exclusive, protective and healing effect on chronic diseases, of which cancer is one." The importance of these products in preventing chronic disorders and cancer can be demonstrated in the low incidence of these diseases in countries where lactic acid-fermented foods are a staple. These countries include Russia, China, Bulgaria and Romania.

Kuhl, a scientific advisor to the European Atomic Energy Commission in Rome, also advocates lactic acid consumption and treatments as a remedy for radiation sickness. He states that diseased cells are more sensitive to ionizing radiation damage than healthy tissues. Kuhl's advice offers new hope for cancer patients who have undergone radiation therapy and are looking for ways of reversing radiation damage. It could also help patients who have had extensive x-rays or x-ray therapy. Kuhl warns against treating cancer patients with radiation therapy, and opposes the irradiation of foodstuffs for the purpose of preservation.

Kuhl's views on healing cancerous growths using lactic acid are supported by other researchers. The remarkable rarity of cancer in Egypt is mentioned by K. H. Bauer in his book *The Cancer Problem*. Bauer notes that in Egypt, lactic acid fermentation is widely practiced with almost all kinds of vegetables. He also found that Arabs drink substantial amounts of sour milk. And, of course, lactic acid-fermented yogurt, kefir and sourdough breads are also consumed in great quantity. For all these reasons, Kuhl strongly advises eating lactic acid-fermented foods.

The Treatment of Polyps

An example of the powerful healing effect of lactic acid-fermented products can be seen in the treatment of polyps, often associated with cancerous growths. After four to six weeks of intensive ingestion of lactic acid-fermented vegetables, polyps will disappear. A recurrence of the polyps will be unlikely if these fermented vegetables continue to be a staple in the regular diet. Dr. Johannes Kuhl, author of *Checkmate to Cancer*, has observed this treatment first hand, and recommends that anyone suffering from polyps should try it. He feels very strongly that every effort should be made to make lactic acid-fermented products a dietary staple. Dr. Kuhl believes that if this were the case, the incidences of cancer would decrease substantially.

Superior and Inferior Lactic Acids

Lactic acid fermentation gives rise to two different forms of lactic acid: L(+) and D(-) lactic acid. Lactic acid-fermented foods like sauerkraut contain more of the L(+) acid which, happily, is the physiologically superior form because it corresponds to the human metabolism.

First and foremost, L(+) lactic acid is necessary for the creation of energy in the muscles, liver and red blood cells. It becomes one of the base substances for making glucose, fatty acids and hormones-things the body needs continuously for health and survival. And, while the body can make its own lactic acid, supplementing our diets with foods rich in L(+) lactic acid has many positive effects on our metabolism.

The latest scientific research suggests that D(-) lactic acid, under conditions of normal ingestion, does not present a burden to the human metabolism. Nevertheless, many authorities state that tumor cells and disturbed intestinal flora produce mainly D(-) lactic acid. The appearance of D(-) lactic acid inside the human metabolism must therefore be considered a sign of metabolic disturbance.

D(-) lactic acid build-up is often blamed for muscle aches and cramps. While there is a correlation between them, it must be made clear that D(-) lactic acid in the muscles is usually produced during hard aerobic activity when there is insufficient oxygen coming from the blood to the muscles. Oxygen is necessary to metabolize pyruvic acid (a "good acid") and, in extreme aerobic conditions, the available oxygen is insufficient to meet the needs of the contracting muscles. The result is that pyruvic acid is converted to D(-) lactic acid. When this happens, the muscles begin to ache or even cramp due to the build-up of lactic acid in the muscle fibers. Not to worry, however, with enough rest, and intake of carbohydrate-rich foods, the cramps or tightness will soon go away.

Medical evidence assures us that L(+) lactic acid is preferred as a food source. Lactic acid-fermented sauerkraut contains mainly this type of acid.

The Healing Power of Cabbage

With the advent of new methods of treating disease, the healing power of cabbage was often overlooked. Today, however, the healing benefits of cabbage are being rediscovered. Various skin diseases respond well to cabbage poultices (mashed leaves or sauerkraut). Intestinal diseases have been successfully treated with cabbage, as have fever and rheumatic pains. Tumors have been reduced with cabbage applications from within and without. The beautiful thing about treatment with cabbage is that it is totally natural and without any side-effects.

According to herbalist and botanist Camille Droz, a poultice of cabbage leaves augments the secretions of festering wounds and inflamed skin tissues, and penetrates healthy skin to heal diseased tissue underneath.

Droz also recommends an application of cabbage leaves in cases of gangrene and a great number of skin conditions. In his writings he provides numerous proofs for his claims and has published many letters from healed and happy patients. It is remarkable that lactic acid-fermented cabbage as well as raw, crushed or mashed cabbage, offers such great healing powers.

Professor Hartmann, a famous German medical doctor, recommends raw sauerkraut for the cleansing of septic wounds. The well-known German surgeon Professor F. Sauerbruch, who confirmed that surgical wounds healed much quicker and better if patients ate raw sauerkraut during recovery, reinforces this seemingly strange recommendation. The healing action of the lactic acid in the sauerkraut is not surprising given that lactic acid alleviates ailments like hardening of the arteries, rheumatism, gout and liver problems.

Medical doctors have successfully treated asthma, chronic constipation and sciatica with a therapy of several weeks of regular sauerkraut eating. The healing effect of sauerkraut is primarily due to the presence of lactic acid and choline.

Raw sauerkraut juice is an excellent and natural remedy for worms, especially in children suffering from roundworm. It is inexpensive, and healthier than using prescription drugs. It seems that sauerkraut even has bactericidal properties, in particular, against typhoid bacteria, as evidenced by a typhoid fever epidemic in Stuttgart, Germany during 1952-53. Sauerkraut was systematically tested as a possible cause of the epidemic, but it was found that, contrary to being causative, it killed the offending bacteria within six hours, provided the sauerkraut was fresh.

How to make a Cabbage Poultice

Cabbage leaves can be applied externally in cases of soreness and inflammation. The leaves should be cut into strips and applied as a poultice that is renewed mornings and evenings. In acute conditions the leaves will turn brown within a few hours and must be replaced more often. When the leaves turn yellow and dry out, therapy can be considered concluded. The leaves can no longer find toxins to neutralize. (Unfortunately, this effect can also occur if the condition does not respond to cabbage leaf treatment.) External application must be supported by internal treatment as well, i.e., consuming sauerkraut and avoiding sugar and sugary foods, white flour, alcohol and nicotine.

Sauerkraut Home Remedies

In a well-known text on home remedies, Dr. Bernd Jurgens advocates the use of lactic acid-fermented sauerkraut in both health and sickness. He offers the following sound advice on the use of sauerkraut.

Anemia • Daily, one lb (1/2 kg) of lactic acid-fermented sauerkraut eaten in small amounts throughout the day.

Arteriosclerosis • Daily, one lb (1/2 kg) of lactic acid-fermented sauerkraut eaten in small amounts throughout the day and repeated several times a year.

Bronchial asthma • Daily, one lb (1/2 kg) of raw lactic acid-fermented sauerkraut mixed with one raw onion and one raw garlic clove.

Diabetes • Three times daily, 1/2 glass of sauerkraut juice taken 1 1/2 hours before meals, plus, daily, one lb (1/2 kg) of lactic acid-fermented sauerkraut eaten in small amounts throughout the day.

Gout • Daily, one lb (1/2 kg) of lactic acid-fermented sauerkraut eaten in small amounts throughout the day.

Longevity • Daily, one lb (1/2 kg) of lactic acid-fermented sauerkraut eaten in small amounts throughout the day for four weeks at least twice a year.

Rheumatism • Daily, one lb (1/2 kg) of lactic acid-fermented sauerkraut eaten in small amounts throughout the day.

Worms *(roundworm, tapeworm, pinworm, etc.)* • Drink 1/2 glass of sauerkraut juice before each meal and eat 1/2 cup sauerkraut on an empty stomach each morning until the worms are gone for good.

A Final Word . . . .

Whether you incorporate sauerkraut into your diet for preventative or curative reasons—or even if you do it simply because it tastes great, you can do so with the certainty that many body processes and organs will be stimulated and strengthened by the workings of the lactic acid.

This ancient and remarkable food has sustained emperors, explorers and common people for thousands of years. Lactic acid-fermented vegetables prove that we can be well fed and well nourished at once—a rare combination in this age of processed and synthetic foods. Once you have tried the recipes in this book your imagination will leap to the fun task of creating more delicious and healthful dishes of your own. Guten Appetit!

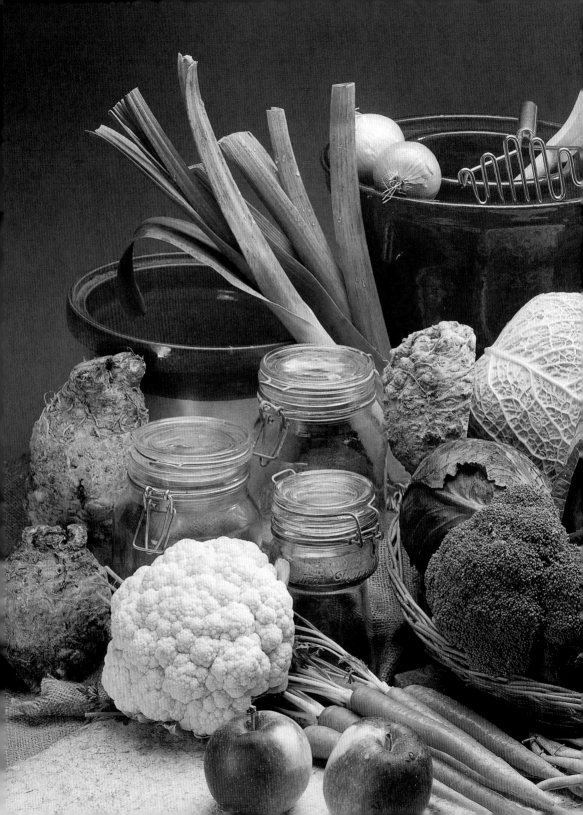

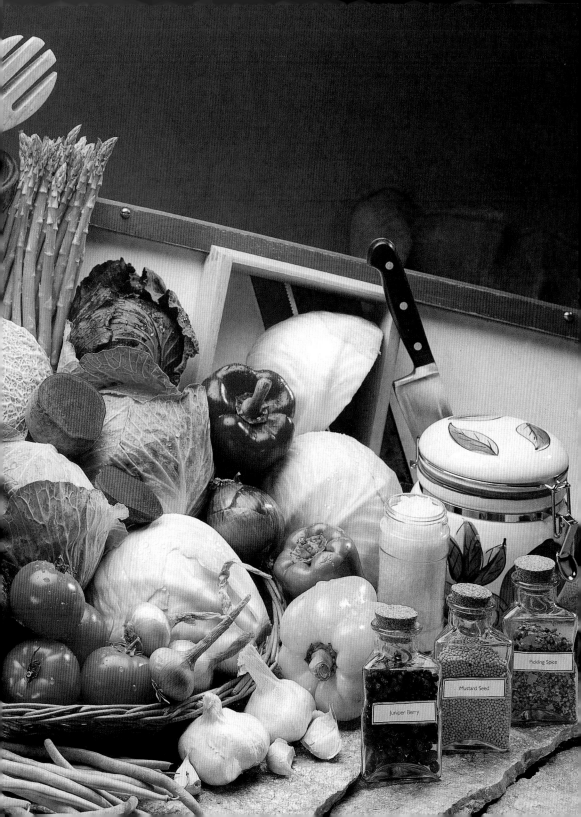

Juniper Berry

Mustard Seed

Pickling Spice

Apple-Sauerkraut Salad
on a Bed of Butter Lettuce

In addition to vitamins, minerals, fiber and lactic acid, you'll get plenty of enzymes from both the sauerkraut and the apple. Aside from the many nutrients, this combination is refreshing and appetizing.

1 large organic apple, cut in segments

1½ cups (375 ml) sauerkraut

1½ cups (375 ml) fennel, julienned

¼ cup (60 ml) walnuts, lightly roasted

¼ cup (60 ml) cold-pressed flax seed oil or extra-virgin olive oil

6 leaves butter lettuce

Place lettuce onto plates. In a bowl, toss together remaining ingredients. Place on top of the lettuce and serve.

Serves 2

Fennel, also known as anise, is a common vegetable in Italian markets. It is a healthy relative of the parsley and adds a mild, sweet flavor to any meal.

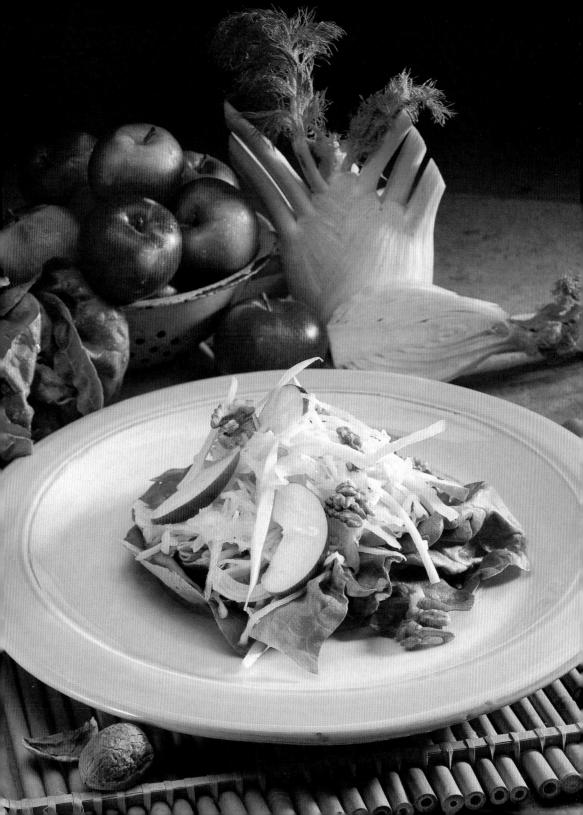

Horseradish Sauerkraut with Grapefruit

The grapefruit adds a delightful citrus flavor in a tangy salad that makes a delicious snack, lunch or dinner. The sharp edge of horseradish opens your sinuses and boosts your circulation.

2 cups (500 ml) sauerkraut

2 pink grapefruit, peeled and segmented

1½ Tbsp horseradish, freshly grated

2 Tbsp green onion, chopped

1½ Tbsp cold-pressed untoasted sesame seed oil

In a bowl, toss together all the ingredients and serve at once.

Serves 2

A member of the mustard family, horseradish owes its kick to its mustard oil content. It is also rich in iron and potassium. Pick up plump, crisp horseradish roots at any Asian market or produce store. Refrigerate and use within one week.

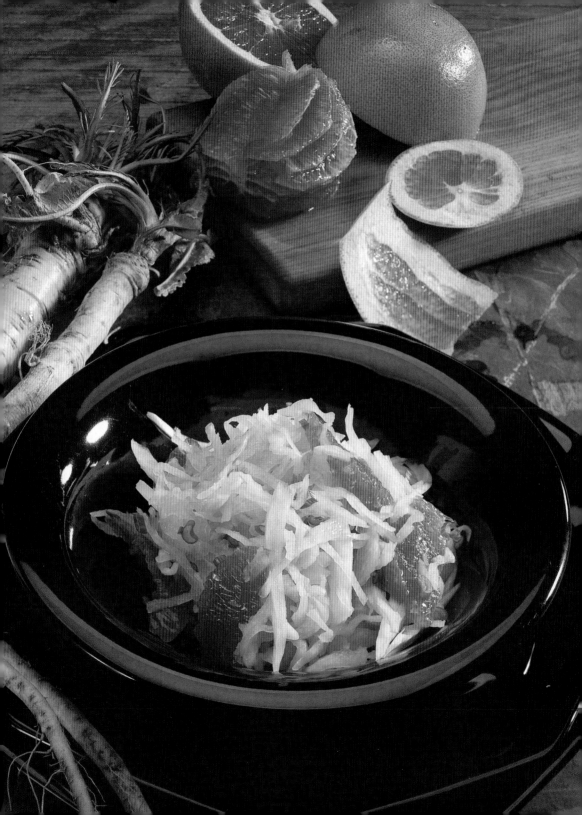

Reuben Sandwich

Famous throughout North America, the Reuben sandwich in fact comes from the Ukraine and Russia. This humble sandwich is delicious any time of year.

4 slices 100% rye bread

2 Tbsp butter

4 slices Swiss Emmenthal cheese

1½ cups (375 ml) sauerkraut

1 large vine-ripened tomato, sliced

3 cups (750 ml) mixed organic salad

1 small red onion, thinly sliced

3 Tbsp cold-pressed flax seed oil

2 Tbsp balsamic vinegar

Vegetable salt such as Herbamare or Spike, to taste

Toast bread and spread with butter. Assemble sandwich by layering in this order: cheese, sauerkraut, tomato and cheese. Cut in half. Toss salad greens and onion with flax seed oil, balsamic vinegar and vegetable salt, and serve with the Reuben.

Serves 2

Good fats make meals tasty and more importantly prevent overeating as they give you a sense of satisfaction. Fat-free diets don't satisfy hunger and lead to snacking, which results in obesity.

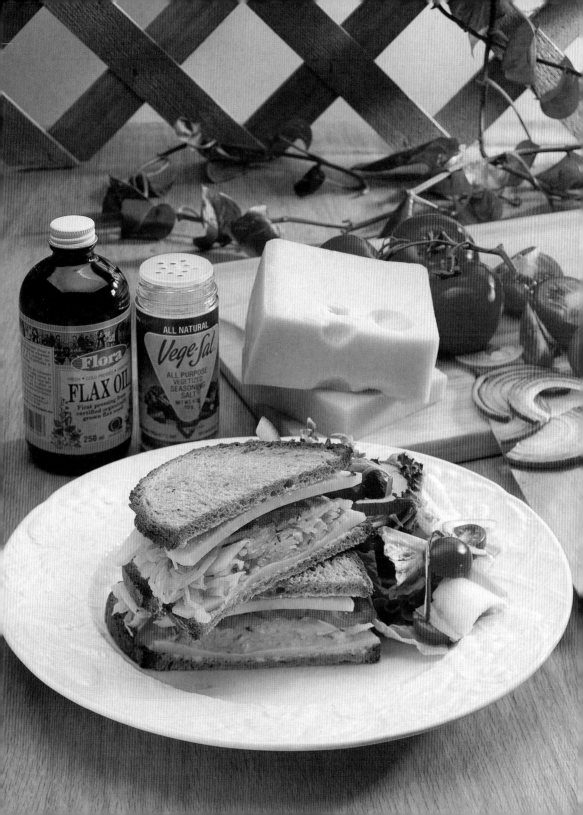

Colorful Sauerkraut Salad

The bright colors and great taste of the salad is sure to please both the eye and the palate. You can serve it with boiled potato or simply with a whole grain baguette.

1 lb (500 g) **green asparagus, tips only**

1 cup (250 ml) **sauerkraut**

1 large yellow bell pepper, thinly sliced

1 large red bell pepper, thinly sliced

½ onion, thinly sliced

4 Tbsp extra-virgin olive oil or cold-pressed flax seed oil

2 Tbsp white balsamic vinegar or apple cider vinegar

2 Tbsp green onion, chopped

Vegetable salt such as Herbamare or Spike, to taste

Place asparagus tips in a pot of boiling water for 1 to 1½ minutes. Remove and rinse with cold water to halt the cooking process and retain the asparagus' bright color. In a bowl, toss sauerkraut, peppers and onion with oil and vinegar. Season with vegetable salt. Sprinkle with green onion and serve.

Serves 2

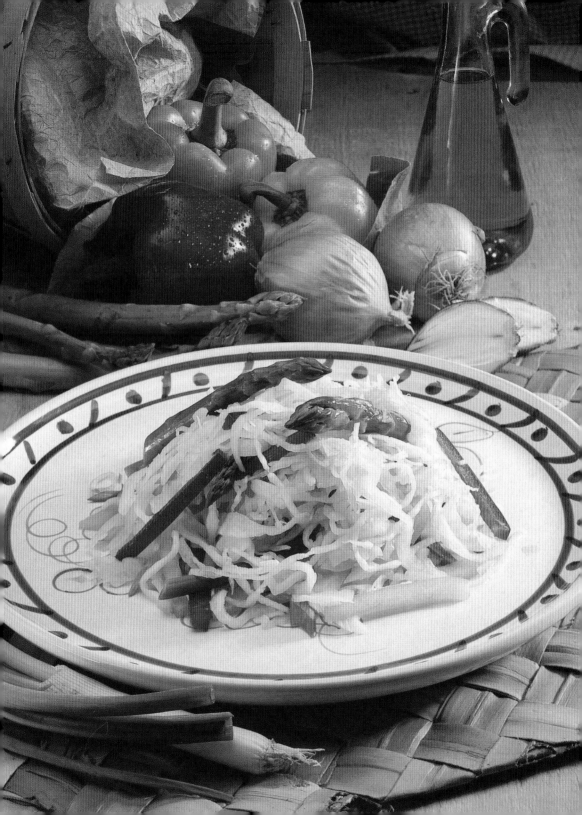

Pineapple Sauerkraut with Roasted Potato

This mouthwatering meal is very popular among vegetarians. Expectant mothers also crave the sauerkraut and pineapple for their health effects and enzymes. The onion is healthful, too—it adds natural antibiotic properties.

2 cups (500 ml) **sauerkraut**

1½ cups (375 ml) **fresh ripe pineapple, cubed**

1 small red onion or Bermuda onion, thinly sliced

2 Tbsp cold-pressed untoasted sesame seed oil

Vegetable salt such as Herbamare or Spike, to taste

1 Tbsp chives, chopped

1½ Tbsp butter

6 medium or 2 cups (500 ml) **Yukon Gold potatoes, diced**

In a pot, cover potatoes with water and boil for 5 to 7 minutes.

In the meantime, mix sauerkraut, pineapple and onion in a bowl. Toss with oil then season with vegetable salt.

Drain potatoes. In a pan, melt butter and toss potatoes until golden. Season with vegetable salt and place on plates with the pineapple sauerkraut. Sprinkle with chives and serve.

Serves 2

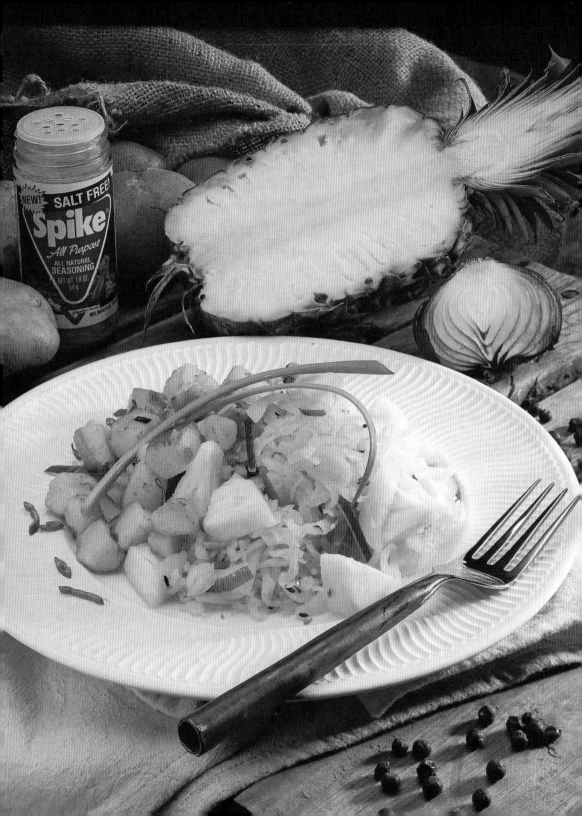

Pickle and Sauerkraut Salad

Simply delicious and refreshing on a hot summer day, both the pickle and sauerkraut replace potassium and sodium lost from the body. Eat the salad as a side dish or snack with pumpernickel or whole grain bread. Seasoning isn't added because all the flavor you need comes from the pickle.

1½ cups (375 ml) **sauerkraut**

1 cup (250 ml) **pickled cucumbers, cubed**

1 **medium-size red or white onion, thinly sliced**

3 Tbsp **cold-pressed flax seed oil**

1 Tbsp **fresh parsley, chopped**

In a bowl, toss together sauerkraut, pickles, onion and oil. Sprinkle with parsley and serve.

Serves 2

[See cucumber recipe on page 22] Fresh, lactic acid-fermented cucumbers with their mild acidity and spicy taste are universal favorites.

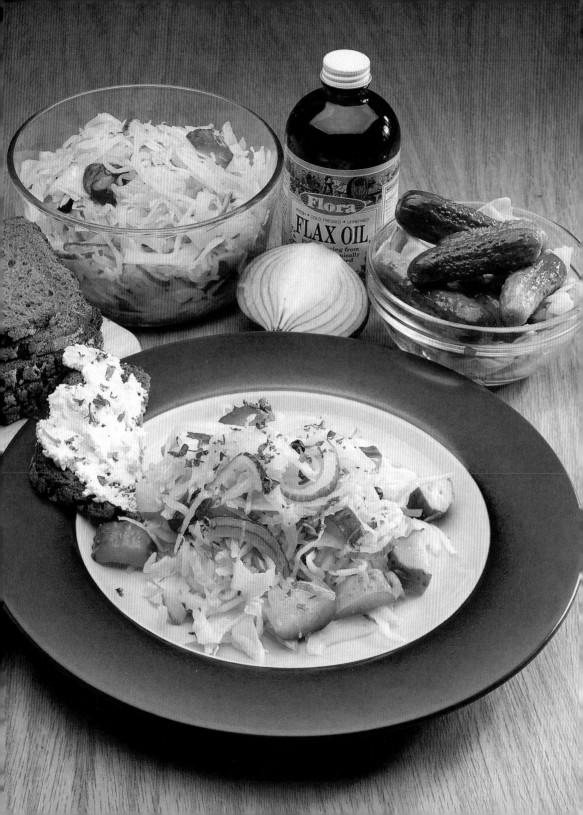

Sauerkraut with Shredded Carrot and Dates

The sweet taste of carrots and dates blends with the sauerkraut in a unique combination. This salad is perfect just before a sports activity such as tennis because it gives you energy and fills you up without being too heavy. Add the jalapeno only if you like it spicy.

2 cups (500 ml) **sauerkraut**

1½ cups (375 ml) **carrots, shredded**

1 cup (250 ml) **dates, sliced**

4 Tbsp cold-pressed walnut or flax seed or pumpkin seed oil

2 medium-size jalapeno peppers, finely chopped (optional)

Mix all ingredients in a bowl and serve.

Serves 2

Carrots contain by far the most beta-carotene–an important antioxidant–of any vegetable. As for the carrot greens, you can use them in cooking just like parsley. In Holland, the leafy fronds were once used by fashion-conscious women as hair decoration.

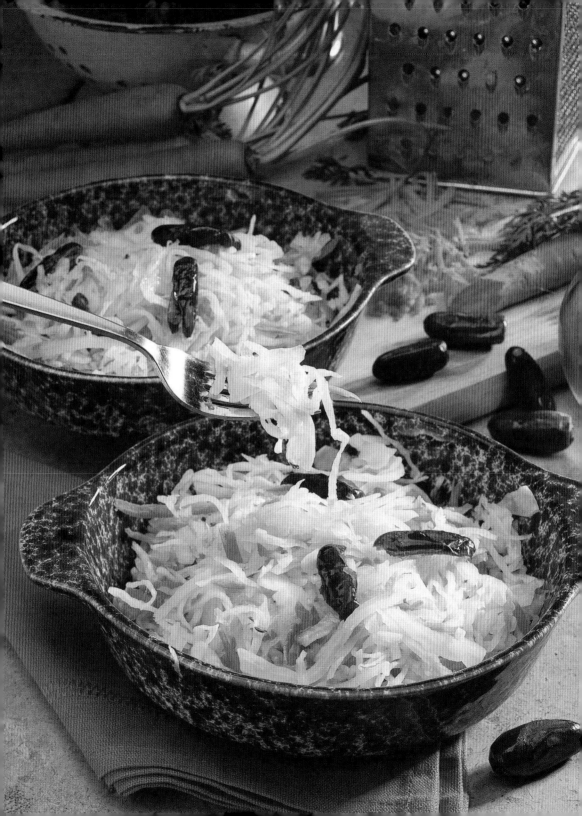

Vegetable Stew with Sauerkraut-Radish Salad

Full of flavor and texture, this hearty stew is an ideal dish for vegans. The sauerkraut-radish salad makes this a completely nourishing meal.

Stew:

1 cup (250 ml) **potato, diced**

2 cups (500 ml) **vegetable stock or water**

1½ cups (375 ml) **green beans, cut in half**

1 cup (250 ml) **onion, julienned**

1 cup (250 ml) **tomatoes, cut in chunks**

3 cloves garlic, chopped

2 bay leaves

1 sprig rosemary, chopped

2 Tbsp extra-virgin olive oil

Vegetable salt such as Herbamare or Spike, to taste

Salad:

1½ cups (375 ml) **sauerkraut**

½ cup (125 ml) **radish, sliced**

1 Tbsp fresh parsley, chopped

2 Tbsp avocado or hazelnut oil

In a medium-size pot, cook potatoes in vegetable stock for 5 to 7 minutes. Add green beans, bay leaf and tomato.

In a separate pan, sauté garlic and onion in oil then add to the pot of potatoes. Cook for 2 minutes longer then stir in rosemary and season with vegetable salt.

In a bowl, toss sauerkraut, radish and parsley with the oil. Serve at once with the stew.

Serves 2

Parsley is an excellent source of iron and vitamins A, B and C. It is said to strengthen the adrenal glands and aid digestion, particularly the digestion of fats. Stir it into soups and stews and use it liberally in salads. For a fresh supply, grow your own—parsley will thrive year-round on a sunny windowsill.

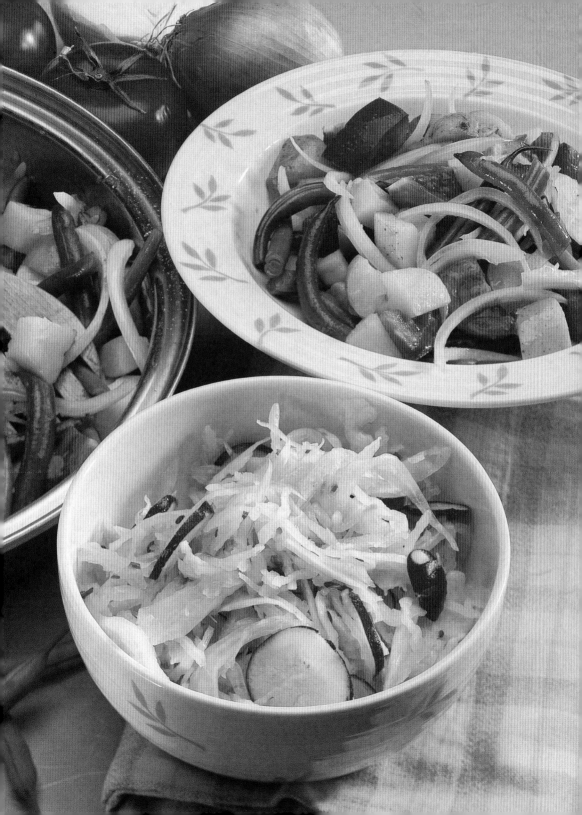

Kalamata and Sauerkraut
with Oven-Roasted Potatoes

Make yourself a tasty and satisfying meal with this versatile combination. Add any kind of garden vegetable to the potatoes to make it more hardy, for instance, zucchini, eggplant, tomato or leek.

6 medium-size or 2 cups (500 ml) Yukon Gold potatoes, cut in half

4 Tbsp extra-virgin olive oil

2 cloves garlic, minced

½ Tbsp + ½ Tbsp fresh herbs such as rosemary, cilantro and tarragon, chopped

1½ cups (375 ml) sauerkraut

1 small red onion, thinly sliced

½ cup (125 ml) Kalamata olives

2 Tbsp butter

Toss potato in oil, garlic and herbs. Bake in the oven for 25 minutes until golden at 375°F (190°C).

In the meantime, place sauerkraut, onion, olives and herbs onto plates. Melt butter and drizzle overtop. Serve with oven-roasted potatoes.

Serves 2

Olive oil is an essential part of a healthy diet and is ideal to cook with. The bitter principle in olives, olive oil and olive leaves has antiviral, antibacterial and antiprotozoic properties. If you eat olives and olive oil on a regular basis, you help protect yourself from all kinds of illnesses and infections. Use olive oil for cooking, but keep the temperature below 220°F (106°C) to preserve its nutritional value.

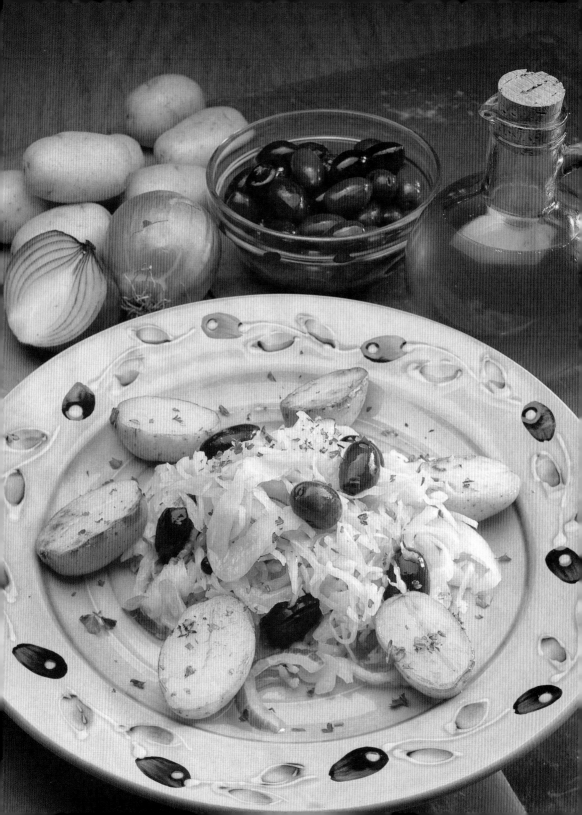

bibliography

Bauer, K. H. *The Cancer Problem.*

Bittere Pillen Autorenteam. *Kursbuch Gesundheits-Fahrplan für ein gesundes Leben.* Germany.

Bruker, Dr. M.O. *Gesund durch richtiges Essen.* Germany: Tomus Verlag.

Droz, Camille. *Von den Wunderbaren Heilwirkungen des Kohlblattes.* Les Geneveys-Sur-Coffrane, Neuenburg, Switzerland, 1985.

Eichholtz, Dr. Fritz. *Die biologische Milchsäure und ihre Entstehung in vegetabilischem Material.* Eden, Germany, 1975.

Jürgens, Dr. Bernd. *Hausrezepte der Naturheilkunde—Eine Sammlung homöopatischer und biologischer Heilmethoden.* Bern and Stuttgart: Hallwag Verlag, 1982.

Kaufmann, Klaus. *Kefir Rediscovered!* Burnaby, BC: alive books, 1997.

Kaufmann, Klaus. *kombucha Rediscovered!* Burnaby, BC: alive books, 1996.

Kuhl, Dr. Johannes. *Biologischer Strahlenschutz: Das milchsaure Getreideschrot—Müsli.* Bern, Switzerland Humata Verlag.

Kuhl, Dr. Johannes. *Krebs und Bestrahlung: Ein Irrtum Moderner Medizin.* Braunlage, Germany: Viadrina Verlag, 1966.

Leibold, Gerhard. *Das große Hausbuch der Natur Heilkunde.* Bassermann, Germany.

Leitzmann, Dr. Claus, and Helmut Million. *Vollwertküche für Genießer: Mit Lust und Liebe.* Germany: Falken Verlag, 1991.

Locher, Hans-Rudolf, and H. L. Friedrich. *Lehm/Moor/ Kohlblatt.* Zürich, Switzerland: Verlag Volks-gesundheit.

Luh, Bor Shiun and Jasper Guy Woodroof. *Commercial Vegetable Processing.* 2nd ed. New York: Avi Book.

Prescott, S.C., C.G. Dunn and Cecil Gordon. *Prescott and Dunn's Industrial Microbiology.* Westport, CT: Avi Pub., 1982.

Schneider, Dr. E. *Nutze die Heilkraft unserer Nahrung.* Hamburg, Germany: Saatkorn-Verlag, 1985.

Schöneck, Annelies. *Making Sauerkraut and Pickled Vegetables at Home.* Burnaby, BC: alive books, 1988.

Stanbury, P. F. and A. Whitaker. *Principles of Fermentation Technology.* Oxford, England: Pergamon Press, 1987.

Stirnimann, Beat. *Sauerkraut als Delikatesse Entdeckt.* Aarau, Switzerland: AT Verlag, 1988.

Taber, Clarence Wilbur. *Taber's Cyclopedic Medical Dictionary.* 17th ed. Philadelphia: F.A. Davis Co., 1989.

Trenev, Natasha, and Leon Chaitow, ND. *Probiotics: The Revolutionary Friendly Bacteria Way to Vital Health and Well-Being.* Wellingborough, England: Thorsons Publishing Group, 1990.

Trum Hunter, Beatrice. *Fermented Foods and Beverages: An Old Tradition.* New Canaan, CT: Keats, 1973.

Vonarburg, Bruno. *Gottes Segen in der Natur.* Stein am Rhein, Germany: Christiana-Verlag, 1977.

Weber, Marlis, and Isabel Wilden. *Lexikon der Gesunden Ernährung.* Germany: Hädecke Gesundheit, 1991.

Whitaker, John R. *Food Related Enzymes.* Washington, DC: American Chemical Society, 1974.

sources

for further education in Natural Heath & Nutrition:
Alive Academy of Natural Health
Ste. 100
12751 Vulcan Way
Richmond, BC V6V 3C8
Canada
Tel: 604-435-1919 or 1-800-663-6580
www.aliveacademy.com

the fermentation crock with the airlock feature mentioned in this book is available at:
Alpha Health Products
7434 Fraser Park Dr.
Burnaby, BC V5J 5B9
Canada
Tel: 604-436-0545 or 1-800-663-2212
Fax: 6004-435-4862
www.alphahealth.ca
Also available from Alpha Health Products are juicers, cabbage shredders for making sauerkraut, Kefir cultures, as well as other health related products.

Remedies and supplements mentioned in this book are available at quality health food stores and nutrition centres.

Acknowledgements

The main credit belongs to Annelies Schöneck, who is the sole author of the original *Making Sauerkraut and Pickled Vegetables at Home*, on which this book is based. May sauerkraut be the blessed vegetable of choice on every plate at least once a week.

Published by Books Alive
PO Box 99
Summertown, TN 38483
(931) 964-3571
(888) 260-8458
www.bookpubco.com

Copyright© 1997, 2008 by Klaus Kaufmann and Annelies Schöneck

Book Design: Paul Chau

Artwork: Terence Yeung
          Guy Andrews

Cover & Inside Photos:
  Edmond Fong, Siegfried Gursche

Recipes & Food Styling: Fred Edrissi

Photo Editing:
  Sabine Edrissi-Bredenbrock

Proofreading: Julie Cheng

The Library of Congress has already cataloged an earlier printing under the publisher name "Alive Books" as follows:

Library of Congress Cataloging-in-Publication Data

Kaufmann, Klaus.

  Making sauerkraut and pickled vegetables at home : creative recipes for lactic-fermented food to improve your health / Klaus Kaufmann and Annelies Schøneck.

    p. cm.

  Includes bibliographical references and index.

  ISBN 978-1-55312-037-7

  1. Fermented foods. 2. Fermented foods--Therapeutic use. 3. Sauerkraut. 4. Sauerkraut--Therapeutic use. I. Schøneck, Annelies. II. Title.

  TP371.44.K387 2007   664'.024--dc22
                  2007001496

ISBN 978-1-55312-037-7

Printed in Hong Kong

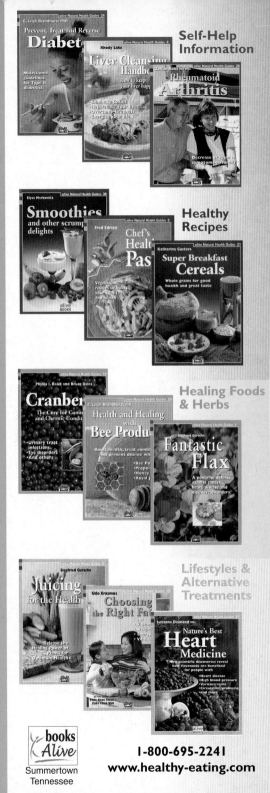

Self-Help Information

Healthy Recipes

Healing Foods & Herbs

Lifestyles & Alternative Treatments

alive Natural Health Guides

About these authors ....

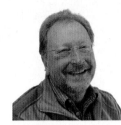

Klaus Kaufmann is an internationally recognized scientific writer, holistic life science counsellor, lecturer and eco-trophologist at the alive Academy of Nutition in Burnaby, BC. Kaufmann is also studying for a Doctor of Science degree.

Annelies Schöneck was born in Germany in 1920. After completing a teaching degree in farming economy, she moved to Sweden in 1953. Since then she has accumulated a vast knowledge of human nutrition and become a pioneer in the cultivation and refinement of natural lactic acid fermented foods.

Through her related publications, seminars, and workshops, Annelies has reached a worldwide audience. Her books on the natural lactic acid fermentation of vegetables, including this revised edition of *Making Sauerkraut and Pickled Vegetables at Home*, have been translated into several languages.

Other books in by Klaus Kaufmann:

Silica: The Amazing Gel
Silica: The Forgotten Nutrient
Devil's Claw Root
The Joy of Juice Fasting
Eliminating Poison in Your Mouth
Kombucha Rediscovered!
Kefir Rediscovered!

About this series ....

The **Alive Natural Health Guides** is the first series of its kind in North America. Each book focuses on a specific natural health related topic and explains how you can improve your health and lifestyle through diet and natural healing methods.

books Alive
Summertown
Tennessee

1-800-695-2241
www.healthy-eating.com